# GUT HEALTH COOKBOOK

Complete Guide On Recipes To Promote A Healthy Gut Microbiome, Including Fermented Foods, Prebiotics, And Probiotics

DR. WAYLON DEBRA

Although it is frequently disregarded in popular debates about nutrition and health, gut health is a vital component of overall well-being. It includes the intricate interactions between many elements in the gastrointestinal tract that impact immune system performance, digestion, nutritional absorption, and even mental health.

The gut microbiome, a complex collection of bacteria that live in the digestive system, is fundamental to gut health. The delicate ecosystem that includes bacteria, fungi, viruses, and other microorganisms is essential to the gut's ability to remain harmonious and in balance. Therefore, dysbiosis, or an imbalance in the gut microbiome, can cause several health problems, including autoimmune diseases, mental health difficulties, and digestive disorders. Therefore, it is crucial to promote general health and well-being by fostering a healthy gut microbiome through dietary and lifestyle choices.

## The Internal Ecosystem of Your Gut Microbiome

The gut microbiome is frequently compared to a thriving city, full of many microbial residents involved in a wide range of metabolic processes. The large intestine is home to the majority of this internal ecosystem, where billions of bacteria collaborate to perform essential tasks that maintain human health.

These include producing vitamins, controlling metabolism, modifying immunological responses, assisting in digestion and nutrition absorption, and even affecting mood and behavior via the gut-brain axis. Several factors, including genetics, diet, lifestyle, drugs, and environmental exposures, affect the composition of the gut microbiome.

A balanced ratio of beneficial to pathogenic microbes and a wide variety of microbial species define a healthy gut microbiome.

It is essential to preserve this variety and balance for both general health and optimum intestinal function.

**Gut Health Is Essential for Overall Well-Being**

Gut health has far-reaching implications for physical, mental, and emotional well-being that go far beyond digestive issues. The efficient digestion and absorption of nutrients, which guarantees that the body gets the necessary vitamins, minerals, and other nutrients for development, repair, and general vigor, depend on a healthy gut flora. Furthermore, the gut microbiome is essential for controlling immune response, acting as a first line of defense against pathogens, and mitigating the risk of autoimmune disorders and inflammatory reactions.

Recent studies have also demonstrated the important role the gut microbiome plays in mental health and cognitive function, with imbalances in the composition of gut microbiota being associated with mood disorders including anxiety and depression. The complex relationship between gut health and mental health is further highlighted by the gut-brain axis, a two-way communication channel between the gut and the brain. To achieve optimal health and vitality, it is crucial to prioritize gut health through dietary treatments and lifestyle alterations.

**Foods Fermented: The Natural Probiotics**

For millennia, humans have included fermented foods in their diets, enjoying their unique tastes and potential health advantages. Natural fermentation is the process by which these traditional foods produce lactic acid, acetic acid, and ethanol.

Beneficial microorganisms like bacteria and yeasts break down sugars and starches in the food substrate.

The food's flavor and texture are improved by the fermentation process, which also boosts the food's nutritional content and encourages the growth of probiotics—beneficial bacteria. Sourdough bread, yogurt, kefir, sauerkraut, kimchi, kombucha, miso, and tempeh are a few examples of fermented foods.

Eating fermented foods can contribute to the diversity and replenishment of the gut microbiome by introducing good bacteria that enhance immunological and digestive health. Fermented foods are also a great complement to a gut-healthy diet because they are full of nutrients and enzymes that help with digestion and absorption of nutrients. Including a range of fermented foods in one's diet can support gut health in general and assist keep the balance of gut bacteria in check.

**Prebiotics: The Microbes' Fuel**

Prebiotics are indigestible fibers that feed good bacteria in the stomach and can be found in some foods. As opposed to probiotics, which are live microorganisms consumed through fermented foods or supplements, prebiotics are organic substances found in nature that promote the expansion and function of good bacteria that are already present in the stomach.

Prebiotics are frequently found in fruits, vegetables, whole grains, legumes, nuts, and seeds; in particular, soluble fiber-rich foods including chicory root, Jerusalem artichokes, onions, garlic, leeks, oats, and bananas are good sources of prebiotics. Prebiotics are ingested and travel through the digestive system undigested until they reach the colon, where they are fermented by gut bacteria to produce butyrate, acetate, and propionate, which are short-chain fatty acids. These fats have been linked to several health advantages, such as a strengthened immune system, decreased inflammation, and improved gut barrier function. They also supply energy to colonocytes, the cells that line the colon. Consuming meals high in prebiotics can help people encourage the growth of gut-healthy bacteria and improve their gut health in general.

**Probiotics: Taking Care of Your Microbiota**

Live bacteria known as probiotics can benefit one's health if consumed in large enough amounts.

These good bacteria live in the gut and influence immunological response, digestion, and general health in different ways. Fermented foods including yogurt, kefir, sauerkraut, kimchi, and kombucha, as well as dietary supplements, naturally contain probiotics. The genera Lactobacillus and Bifidobacterium contain the majority of common probiotic strains, although other strains with possible health advantages have also been researched, including Saccharomyces boulardii, Bacillus coagulans, and several strains of Escherichia coli. Probiotics produce antimicrobial chemicals, modulate immune responses, colonize the gut, compete with pathogenic bacteria for nutrients and adhesion sites, and improve the function of the gut barrier. Probiotics have been shown through clinical research to be effective in treating a range of gastrointestinal conditions, including lactose intolerance, antibiotic-associated diarrhea, inflammatory bowel disease, and irritable bowel syndrome (IBS). Probiotics have also been demonstrated to enhance immune system performance, lower the risk of infection, lessen allergy symptoms, and even enhance mental health results. Probiotic efficacy, however, can differ based on several variables, including the strain(s) utilized, the dosage, the makeup of the user's gut microbiome, and the existence of underlying medical disorders. Therefore, before beginning a probiotic supplementation regimen, make sure to select probiotic products supported by scientific data and speak with a healthcare provider. Through the use of foods and supplements high in probiotics, people can support and maintain the health of their gut microbiota.

## Disclaimer

Waylon Debra Disclaimer the recipes and dietary suggestions presented in this cookbook are intended for informational purposes only and the information provided should not be considered a substitute for professional medical advice, diagnosis, or treatment.

Before making any significant changes to your diet or exercise routine, consult with a qualified healthcare professional.

Individual dietary needs vary, and what may be suitable for one person may not be appropriate for another.

The author and publisher disclaim responsibility for any adverse effects resulting directly or indirectly from the use or application of the information contained in this cookbook.

By using this cookbook, you agree to assume full responsibility for your own health and well-being.

# CHAPTER ONE
## THE BASIS OF HEALTHY COOKING

Writing a cookbook on gut health requires exploring the complex interplay between gut microbiota, nutrition, and general health.

In examining the principles of gut-healthy cooking, it is essential to recognize the critical role the gut microbiota plays in immune response, digestion, and even mental well-being. An in-depth discussion of necessary kitchen supplies, products, and cooking methods that optimize gut health will be covered in this part.

**Essential Kitchen Items for Digestive Health**

Having the appropriate tools and equipment is crucial when it comes to cooking for intestinal health. A well-stocked kitchen not only makes it easier to prepare wholesome meals but also promotes experimenting with different products and cooking techniques. A good blender is a must-have for anybody interested in gut health because it can be used to blend probiotic-rich yogurt or kefir, fruits, and vegetables, as well as other gut-friendly components, to make smoothies. Purchasing a fermentation crock or jars also makes it possible to produce probiotic-rich fermented foods at home, such as kimchi, kombucha, and sauerkraut.

Pots and pans made of stainless steel are better than non-stick ones since they reduce the amount of potentially hazardous chemicals that are present. Storage containers to keep prepared items fresh and easily accessible, as well as sharp blades for easily slicing fibrous vegetables and whole grains, are other kitchen necessities.

By stocking your kitchen with these necessities, you create the foundation for a smooth and joyful cooking experience for gut health.

Knowing Ingredients: Selecting Foods That Are Good for Your Gut

The foundation of any cookbook on gut health is the careful selection of ingredients that support and nurture the complex ecosystem of the gut microbiota. A diet that is favorable to the gut should be based mostly on whole, unprocessed foods since they are rich in fiber and other nutrients that support microbial variety and equilibrium.

Rich in fiber, vitamins, and minerals, leafy greens like spinach, kale, and Swiss chard help maintain digestive health and supply prebiotic fuel for good gut flora.

Including a range of vibrant fruits and vegetables guarantees a varied consumption of antioxidants and phytonutrients, which are essential for lowering inflammation and promoting gut health in general.

Excellent providers of soluble fiber and plant-based protein that support a wholesome gut flora are legumes, beans, and lentils.

Probiotics, or live beneficial bacteria, are abundant in fermented foods like yogurt, kefir, tempeh, and miso and help to improve digestion by promoting the diversity of gut microbes. Incorporating foods high in omega-3, such as walnuts, flaxseeds, and fatty fish, also promotes intestinal integrity and lowers inflammation.

Making these components a priority in your cooking can help you promote good gut health and support your microbiome.

**Cooking Methods to Optimise the Benefits for Gut Health**

Although choosing the right ingredients is crucial, cooking and preparing food has an impact on intestinal health as well. The nutritional integrity of food is preserved by using moderate cooking techniques like steaming, sautéing, and simmering. This keeps important vitamins, minerals, and enzymes that are important for intestinal health. To ensure maximal bioavailability, avoid overheating and extensive cooking durations as these can degrade delicate nutrients.

Soaking or sprouting grains and legumes before cooking might improve their digestibility and lower anti-nutrients like phytic acid, which can impede the absorption of minerals. Including items that have undergone fermentation in your meals improves flavor profiles, aids with digestion, and adds advantageous microorganisms. Adding anti-inflammatory and antibacterial qualities to food, as well as adding depth and complexity, are the benefits of experimenting with herbs and spices like garlic, ginger, and turmeric that promote gut health. Last but not least, adding healthy fats to food—

such as nuts, avocados, and olive oil—improves the absorption of fat-soluble vitamins and maintains the integrity of the intestinal lining. You may maximize the health advantages of gut-friendly ingredients and fully utilize their potential for overall well-being by using these cooking techniques.

# CHAPTER TWO
## FOODS FERMENTED FOR GUT HEALTH

For generations, humans have included fermented foods in their diets, appreciating them not just for their distinct tastes but also for their possible health advantages, especially in supporting a thriving gut microbiota. Food carbs are naturally broken down into acids or alcohol by microbes like bacteria, yeast, or fungi during the fermentation process. By creating helpful components like vitamins, enzymes, and probiotics and boosting the bioavailability of specific nutrients, this procedure not only preserves the food but also improves its nutritional profile.

**Pickles**

Vegetables are one of the most widely consumed types of fermented food.

Fermenting vegetables such as cabbage, cucumbers, carrots, and beets results in savory and nourishing foods.

For instance, shredded cabbage is fermented with salt to make sauerkraut, which promotes the growth of lactic acid bacteria.

These microorganisms contribute to the probiotic content of sauerkraut and give it its sour flavor by converting the carbohydrates in the cabbage into lactic acid. Similar to this, kimchi, a popular Korean dish, is prepared by fermenting a variety of vegetables, including radishes and napa cabbage, with ingredients like garlic, ginger, and chili powder.

The vegetables are a great complement to a diet that promotes gut health because of the fermentation process, which also raises the vegetables' amounts of vitamins, minerals, and good bacteria.

**Fermenting Drinks**

There's another way to include probiotics and other healthy ingredients in your diet: fermented beverages. For example, kombucha is a tart, fizzy beverage derived from fermented tea. It is made by fermenting sweetened tea for a while with a symbiotic culture of bacteria and yeast (SCOBY) added.

The tea's sugars are broken down by the SCOBY during fermentation, creating organic acids, vitamins, and small amounts of alcohol.

The outcome is a revitalizing drink that has probiotic qualities and may aid in promoting intestinal health. Other fermented drinks include kvass, a traditional Slavic beverage prepared from fermented bread or grains, and kefir, a fermented milk drink with Caucasian origins.

These drinks come in a variety of flavors to accommodate a wide range of palates in addition to offering probiotics.

**How to Include Fermented Foods in Your Diet**

Including items that have undergone fermentation in your diet is an easy and delectable method to support gut health. To begin, try a variety of fermented vegetable products, like pickles, kimchi, and sauerkraut, and see which ones you like best.

These can be added to sandwiches, salads, or wraps for an additional flavor and nutritional boost, or they can be eaten as a side dish on their own. Probiotic-rich fermented drinks, such as kefir and kombucha, are a great way to stay hydrated while still getting your nutrients without all the added sugar of sodas or juices.

Additionally, to enhance the nutritional value of your food and give it more depth of flavor, think about cooking with fermented condiments like soy sauce or miso paste.

Include fermented foods daily to support healthy gut bacteria and to take advantage of their delightful flavors and textures.

# CHAPTER THREE
## PREBIOTIC POWERHOUSES

Prebiotics are an important subject when discussing gut health because these food items are essential for promoting the development and activity of good gut bacteria. Prebiotics are essentially indigestible fibers that feed probiotics, which are living bacteria and yeasts that, when taken in sufficient quantities, offer a host of several health benefits. People can effectively promote and maintain a healthy gut microbiome by concentrating on foods high in prebiotics, which can have a good impact on general well-being and health outcomes.

**Examining Prebiotic Foods**

Prebiotic foods are a broad category of plant-based meals that contain particular kinds of fibers, like oligosaccharides, resistant starches, and inulin, which do not break down in the small intestine and instead enter the colon undigested to act as food for good bacteria. Chicory root, garlic, onions, leeks, asparagus, Jerusalem artichokes, bananas, oats, apples, and flaxseeds are a few examples of foods high in prebiotics. These foods contribute to a balanced and robust gut microbiome by not only supplying vital nutrients but also encouraging the growth of advantageous gut bacteria like lactobacilli and bifidobacteria.

**Recipes with Ingredients High in Probiotics**

Prebiotic-rich products can be a tasty and satisfying addition to recipes, improving not just the nutritional value and flavor of food but also supporting intestinal health.

For example, adding roasted garlic to creamy hummus increases the number of prebiotics in the hummus while also adding flavor depth.

In a similar vein, adding oats and flaxseeds to a breakfast smoothie yields a filling and healthy meal that promotes gut health. Furthermore, you may increase the prebiotic content of meals while also adding color, texture, and flavor by adding a variety of prebiotic-rich vegetables, like asparagus, broccoli, and spinach, to stir-fries, salads, and soups.

**Including Prebiotics in Typical Meals**

Long-term support of gut health requires regular meals that include foods high in prebiotics. Meals can have their prebiotic content considerably increased with easy substitutions and additions that don't sacrifice convenience or flavor.

For example, adding cooked and cooled potatoes to salads or using whole-grain pasta in place of normal pasta will raise the resistant starch content and provide prebiotic benefits. Furthermore, the fermentation process of fermented foods like sauerkraut or kimchi increases the number of prebiotics in meals in addition to adding probiotics. People can proactively promote their general well-being and gut health by including a variety of prebiotic-rich foods in their regular meals and choosing carefully which ingredients to use.

# CHAPTER FOUR
## HYPOTHETICAL ENCHANTMENTS

Probiotics, also known as "friendly" or "good" bacteria, are essential for preserving a balanced gut microbiome. This section will discuss the role that probiotics play in supporting gut health and will look at how you can include them in your diet by making probiotic-rich dishes and homemade probiotic foods.

**Overview of Probiotics**

Probiotics are live bacteria that give the host health advantages when taken in sufficient doses. These good bacteria mostly live in the stomach and support healthy digestion, immune system performance, and nutrient absorption. Probiotic strains of Lactobacillus, Bifidobacterium, and

Saccharomyces boulardii are among the most popular types.

According to research, preserving a balanced and diverse gut microbiota is essential for good health. But the natural balance of gut bacteria can be upset by several things, including the use of antibiotics, eating poorly, stress, and exposure to environmental toxins. This condition is known as dysbiosis, and it is linked to several gastrointestinal problems as well as immune dysfunction.

Including foods high in probiotics in your diet is a good method to help maintain gut health and microbial balance. Live cultures of healthy bacteria found in these foods colonize the gut and support the restoration of the microbiome. Yoghurt, kefir, sauerkraut, kimchi, miso, tempeh, and kombucha are a few foods high in probiotics.

You can support a healthy gut microbiome and improve general health and well-being by realizing the benefits of probiotics and adding them to your regular meals.

**Creating Beneficial Bacteria at Home with Probiotic Foods**

Making your probiotic foods is an affordable and flexible way to add good bacteria to your diet. You can ensure optimal potency and freshness by controlling the ingredients, fermentation process, and flavor profiles when you cultivate these foods at home.

Yoghurt, which can be made with milk and a starter culture containing live bacterial strains like Lactobacillus bulgaricus and Streptococcus thermophilus, is one of the easiest homemade probiotic foods. Yogurt that has been fermented at a regulated temperature using these cultures is high in calcium, protein, and probiotics.

Similar to this, fermented veggies like kimchi and sauerkraut are simple to prepare at home and offer a powerful probiotic and nutritional boost. Shredded cabbage or other vegetables can be preserved and their flavor and probiotic content increased by simply fermenting them with salt and spices. This process promotes the growth of lactic acid bacteria, which turn sugars into lactic acid.

Kefir, a fermented dairy beverage made by inoculating milk with kefir grains containing a symbiotic culture of yeast and bacteria, and kombucha, an astringent, bubbly tea fermented with a SCOBY (symbiotic culture of bacteria and yeast), are two more homemade probiotic foods. These drinks give you a refreshing way to get your probiotics in while also supporting your immune system and improving your digestion.

By experimenting with various recipes and fermentation methods, you can customize homemade probiotic foods to fit your dietary requirements and taste preferences.

Cultivating good bacteria at home is a gratifying and nourishing experience that supports gut health and overall wellness, whether you're making yogurt, sauerkraut, kefir, or kombucha.

**Probiotic-Packed Foods for Digestive Health**

Including foods high in probiotics in your diet is a tasty and practical approach to improving your general health and gut health. There are a plethora of recipes that support a healthy gut microbiome and include probiotic ingredients, from breakfast to dinner.

Have a probiotic-rich smoothie for breakfast consisting of yogurt or kefir, fresh fruit, leafy greens, and a dash of prebiotic-rich oats or flaxseeds to kickstart your day. This nutrient-dense drink gives you a boost of flavor and a variety of good bacteria and fiber to get you through the day.

Savor a vibrant salad with fermented veggies, such as kimchi or sauerkraut, for lunch. You can also add grilled tempeh or tofu for extra protein and probiotics. Serve it with kombucha or miso soup on the side for a filling, gut-friendly dinner that boosts immunity and digestion.

Make your pizza at dinner with a sourdough crust and probiotic-rich toppings like artichokes, fermented cheese, and olives to include probiotics into your main courses. Serve it with a probiotic-rich side dish like fermented slaw or pickled vegetables, or with a side salad dressed with a kefir-based dressing.

By adding probiotic ingredients, snacks, and desserts can be made into treats that are good for the gut. For a rich and nutritious treat, try a probiotic-rich yogurt parfait topped with layers of fresh fruit and granola or probiotic-rich dark chocolate truffles infused with a hint of kombucha.

Your gut microbiota can be nourished and optimal digestive health and wellness can be promoted by including probiotic-rich dishes in your daily meals. Try out various recipes and flavor combos to find new favorites and savor the mouthwatering advantages of probiotics.

# CHAPTER FIVE
## GUT-HEALTHY BREAKFASTS

A greater understanding of the critical role gut health plays in general well-being has emerged in recent years. More focus is being placed on what we eat and how it affects our gut due to new research that illuminates the complex relationship between the gut microbiome and several aspects of health, such as immune function, mental health, and digestion. Because of this, the idea of a cookbook for gut health has become popular, providing people with a wealth of recipes created specially to support a healthy gut microbiome. Breakfast is a great time to start the day with foods that support and nourish gut health, as it's often regarded as the most significant meal of the day. This section highlights breakfast options that are specifically designed to improve gut health. These include breakfast bowls and smoothies, baked goods that support the gut, and energizing morning openers.

## Activating Morning Commencements

Our mood and behavior throughout the morning are largely determined by the first meal of the day. Energizing morning starters are made to boost intestinal health and give you a quick energy boost. These breakfast options are generally high in fiber, vitamins, and minerals—all of which are critical for supporting the health of the gut flora. For example, adding different toppings to your overnight oats, including berries, almonds, and seeds, not only makes for a quick breakfast but also offers a wide range of nutrients that support healthy gut flora. Similar to this, avocado toast on whole-grain bread is a well-liked option that boosts digestive health and satisfies hunger by combining fiber and healthy fats. Other energizing breakfast options include Greek yogurt parfait with layers of fruit and granola, which offers a combination of probiotics and prebiotics to support gut flora, or chia seed pudding, which is rich in fiber and omega-3 fatty acids. People can optimize their digestive health and feed their bodies for the day by beginning their day with nutrient-dense, gut-friendly foods.

**Smoothies and Bowls for Breakfast**

Smoothies and Bowls for Breakfast

provide an easy and adaptable approach to include a range of gut-healthy nutrients in one meal. Those with hectic schedules who are looking for quick yet wholesome breakfast options may find these options very attractive. A quality breakfast bowl should include a basis of complete grains, like brown rice or quinoa, and be topped with a variety of vegetables, lean meats, and fermented foods, like sauerkraut or kimchi. Poached egg and smoked salmon give more protein and omega-3 fatty acids to a dish, making it more balanced and filling. However, there are countless ways to include components that are good for the gut, such as fruits, yogurt, kefir, and leafy greens, in smoothies. Probiotics like kefir or yogurt increase the health benefits of the smoothie, and other ingredients like avocado, spinach, or kale add vital nutrients and fiber. If you're looking for something sweeter, adding fruits like bananas or berries can naturally sweeten it and offer more fiber. Breakfast bowls and smoothies provide a tasty and easy method to improve intestinal health while satisfying individual taste preferences by mixing a variety of healthful ingredients.

**Digestive-Soothing Pastries**

Although baked goods aren't generally associated with gut health, you may make them more nutritious by adding components that support gut health. Refined flour and sugars, which are frequently included in traditional baked products, can upset gut flora and increase inflammation.

But baked products may be reimagined to promote digestive health with a few easy changes and substitutions. For instance, substituting whole-grain flour like oat flour or almond flour for refined flour offers vital minerals like vitamins B and E along with more fiber. Similar to this, replacing refined sugars with natural sweeteners like honey or maple syrup increases the number of important enzymes and antioxidants while lowering the glycemic load. In addition to adding fiber, adding ingredients like chia or ground flaxseeds to baked products also gives lignans and omega-3 fatty acids, which promote gut health and reduce inflammation. Probiotics are also introduced when fermented foods, such as yogurt or sourdough starter, are used in baked recipes. These meals can aid in better digestion and nutritional absorption.

Through the incorporation of gut-boosting components into classic baked products, people may indulge in their favorite sweets while also promoting gut health and a healthy microbiome.

 breakfast is critical for gut health, and including gut-healthy breakfast options in one's routine can have significant positive effects on general health. There are many ways to improve digestive health and nourish the gut microbiota first thing in the morning, including gut-boosting baked goods, nutrient-packed breakfast bowls and smoothies, and energizing morning starts. People can actively improve their gut health and experience bright, long-lasting wellness by embracing these scrumptious and nourishing breakfast options.

# CHAPTER SIX
## NOURISHING LUNCHES AND DINNERS

Lunches and dinners are crucial when it comes to making nutritional choices that support intestinal health. These meals are a great way to combine foods and cuisines that are expressly meant to support a healthy gut flora, in addition to serving as a source of nourishment. Such meals can make a big difference in overall digestive wellness because they emphasize complete foods, nutritional balance, and gut-friendly components.

Healthy Soups & Stews:

Cooking adaptable foods like soups and stews is a great way to support gut health. They present an excellent chance to include a variety of components that are good for gut health, like veggies, legumes, whole grains, and lean proteins. Additionally, the slow simmering method used to prepare soups and stews aids in the breakdown of nutrients, improving nutrient absorption and making them easier to digest. Add-ins with anti-inflammatory and prebiotic qualities, such as garlic, onions, ginger, and turmeric, can further improve gut health. Furthermore, adding bone broth, which is high in collagen and amino acids, can enhance overall digestive function and promote the integrity of the gut lining.

Bright Salads and Vinegar:

Salads are frequently thought of as the best choice for people looking for a filling and light dinner. When prepared with care, salads can be extremely gut-nourishing. Salads are transformed into nutrient-dense powerhouses by adding a range of leafy greens, vibrant veggies, fruits, nuts, seeds, and fermented foods. Rich in fiber, vitamins, and minerals, leafy greens like spinach, kale, and rocket promote healthy digestive systems. Probiotics are introduced into the diet through fermented foods like sauerkraut, kimchi, and pickles, which help to maintain a healthy gut microbiota. Furthermore, in addition to adding flavor, homemade dressings made with components like olive oil, apple cider vinegar, lemon juice, and herbs also supply important fatty acids and antioxidants that promote gut health.

**Main Courses for Gut Healing:**

The focal point of any lunch or dinner arrangement is the main course, and when prepared with gut health in mind, it can act as a pillar for supporting digestive wellbeing. Adding foods recognized for their ability to heal the gut can turn everyday meals into healing experiences. Lean proteins, like chicken, fish, and tofu, for instance, provide a rich source of the amino acids needed for tissue upkeep and repair. When these proteins are combined with whole grains like buckwheat, brown rice, or quinoa, a good amount of fiber is provided, promoting regular bowel movements and nourishing good bacteria in the stomach. Furthermore, adding fermented foods like miso or tempeh to main courses delivers probiotics that support a balanced gut flora in addition to adding depth of flavor. Additionally, cooking techniques like steaming, baking, or grilling that maintain the nutritional value of ingredients guarantee that the meals maintain their gut-friendly benefits without sacrificing flavor or texture.

# CHAPTER SEVEN
## SNACKS AND SIDES FOR GUT HEALTH

Our regular diets must include snacks and sides because they offer us the chance to include essential nutrients that promote gut health.

It's crucial to provide a range of snack and side dish alternatives in a gut health cookbook that not only tempt the palate but also support a healthy gut microbiota. This area will cover savory and sweet side dishes, nutrient-dense snack options, and gut-friendly spreads and dips that use fermented foods, prebiotics, and probiotics to support healthy gut flora.

**Ideas for Nutrient-Rich Snacks:**

Many people snack frequently throughout the day, and if you make the correct decisions, snacking may be a great way to improve gut health.

A gut health cookbook's nutrient-dense snack suggestion should emphasize using foods high in fiber, probiotics, and prebiotics.

Snack dishes can incorporate fermented foods, such as kimchi, sauerkraut, and kombucha, which offer a boost of good bacteria to promote digestive health. Probiotic-rich foods like yogurt or kefir and foods high in prebiotics like bananas, oats, and flaxseeds can also be enjoyed as snacks.

Additionally, nuts and seeds are great sources of healthy fats, protein, and fiber that support gut health and satiety, making them great as gut-friendly snacks. A gut health cookbook with a range of nutrient-dense snack options can make it simple for people to incorporate foods that support gut health into their daily routine, which in turn promotes a thriving microbiome and general well-being.

**Sweet & Savoury Side Dishes:**

Side dishes are adaptable parts of every meal that, when prepared with gut health in mind, can greatly improve digestive well-being in general. Whole grains, legumes, and cruciferous vegetables are just a few of the savory side dishes that can be included in a gut health cookbook.

These components are high in fiber and vital nutrients that help maintain a healthy gut microbiota. For instance, a robust and nourishing side dish full of components that are good for the gut can be lentil soup with spinach and turmeric or quinoa salad with roasted vegetables.

On the sweeter side, adding antioxidant- and fiber-rich fruits like berries to side dishes like fruit salads or yogurt parfaits can be a tasty way to satiate cravings for sweets and promote gut health. Through the thoughtful balancing of savory and sweet side dishes included in gut health cookbooks, people may nurture their microbiome with each meal and savor a wide variety of flavors.

**Digestible Spreads and Dips:**

Spreads and dips are a great complement to any cookbook on gut health because they provide a practical means of adding items that are good for the gut to snacks and meals. Selecting products that support healthy gut microbiota is crucial when making dips and spreads with digestive wellness in mind. Herb- and spice-infused Greek yogurt dips offer more than just tang and flavor; they also contain probiotics that help maintain digestive health. Another great option for a gut-friendly dip is hummus, which is prepared from chickpeas, tahini, and olive oil. Hummus provides a combination of fiber, protein, and healthy fats. Furthermore, adding fermented foods like tempeh or miso to spreads can boost probiotics and give meals a distinct umami flavor.

These spreads and dips become even more nutritious when paired with sprouted bread, whole-grain crackers, or raw veggies. This makes for filling appetizers and snacks that also support digestive health. A gut-healthy cookbook featuring an assortment of dips and spreads can help people enhance their culinary adventures while providing their bodies with internal nourishment.

# CHAPTER EIGHT
## GUT HAPPINESS DELICACIES

In culinary culture, desserts have a special place and are frequently connected to pleasure and excess. However, conventional desserts that are high in harmful fats and refined sugars may not support the development of a balanced microbiome when it comes to gut health.

A new generation of dessert recipes that are designed to promote digestive health without sacrificing flavor or satisfaction has surfaced in response to this worry. These desserts incorporate elements that are important for supporting a healthy gut flora, together with prebiotics and probiotics. Desserts that contain fermented foods, probiotic sources, and prebiotic-rich components allow people to satisfy their sweet desires without jeopardizing their digestive health.

**Sweets with a Gut-Healthy Experiment:**

This dessert category features classic sugary confections that are transformed into delicious foods that are good for the stomach. Traditional sweets such as cakes, cookies, and muffins are reimagined with gut-healthy components.

For example, recipes may call for whole grain flour, like oat flour or almond flour, which are richer in fiber and have prebiotic benefits, in place of refined flour. Sweeteners like honey or maple syrup can take the place of processed sweets, adding healthy nutrients and a more natural sweetness. Furthermore, fruits, nuts, and seeds are common ingredients in these desserts; these additions not only improve flavor and texture but also add a variety of nutrients that support digestive health. These sweets provide a guilt-free approach to satiate appetites while supporting gut microbiota health by focusing on healthful ingredients and making simple alternatives.

**Desserts Using Ingredients Including Probiotics:**

Live bacteria renowned for their ability to support gut health are called probiotics, and when taken in sufficient quantities, they offer a host of advantages. Desserts with probiotic components help to enhance digestive well-being by utilizing the power of these helpful bacteria.

A popular source of probiotics, yogurt is a main component in many of these sweets. Yogurt gives a rich and creamy texture and a probiotic boost when it's used for creamy parfaits, frozen yogurt desserts, or tangy cheesecakes.

Dessert recipes may also include other fermented foods like miso, kefir, and kombucha, which provide a variety of good bacteria strains to enhance gut diversity. Not only do these sweets offer a tasty way to consume foods high in probiotics, but they also provide a practical approach to adding these healthy bacteria to regular diets.

**Luxurious and Nutritious Treats:**

Desserts are usually thought of as indulgent, but you can make rich desserts that are also good for your stomach. Rich but healthful treats emphasize components that promote digestive well-being without compromising taste or satiety.

For instance, dark chocolate is praised for having antioxidants and is sometimes used in desserts like almond flour brownies or chocolate avocado mousse. Rich in fiber and healthy fats, avocado is a nutrient-dense fruit that gives sweets a creamy, multifaceted texture and prebiotic advantages. Nut butter—which can be produced from peanuts, cashews, or almonds—provides a source of protein and healthy fats while also adding to their pleasing texture and flavor. Indulgent desserts can become a part of a gut-friendly lifestyle that supports general well-being by combining these healthful components with careful portion proportions and a balanced diet.

sweets that support gut health provide a tasty and fulfilling way to assist digestive wellness. These sugary delights offer a guilt-free enjoyment that nourishes the body from the inside out by combining ingredients high in probiotics, prebiotics, and other nutrients crucial for gut health. Indulging in sweets with a gut-healthy twist, probiotic-infused pastries, or rich yet nutritional treats—there are a plethora of methods to fulfill appetites without sacrificing digestive health. Dessert time may become an occasion to celebrate gut happiness and flavor with a little imagination and thoughtful ingredient selection.

Drinks are important for gut health since they can either make digestion uncomfortable or encourage a healthy microbiota. In this episode, we'll examine the wide range of drinks made to promote gut health, including their components, advantages, and possible effects on digestive health.

**Drinks that Refresh and Have Gut-Friendly Flavours:**

Not only may refreshing drinks quench your thirst, but they can also contain a lot of substances that are good for your gut. Gut-friendly flavors like ginger, lemon, and mint can add a pleasant edge to beverages while also helping with digestion.

Renowned for its anti-inflammatory qualities, ginger facilitates food passage through the digestive tract and eases symptoms of nausea and indigestion. Citrus fruits like lemons, which are high in vitamin C, not only provide food with a refreshing taste but also help the body produce digestive fluids that aid in the absorption of nutrients. Mint is also well-known for its calming qualities, which can aid in promoting digestion and easing gastrointestinal discomfort. People can enjoy a delicious method to promote their gut health by adding these items to smoothies, herbal teas, and infused water.

**Teas & Infusions for Healing:**

For ages, people have been drinking tea because of its many health benefits, which include supporting digestive health. A natural and gentle approach to support gut health is through the use of healing teas and infusions, which are produced from a range of herbs, spices, and botanicals.

For example, chamomile tea is well-known for its relaxing effects on the digestive tract, which makes it a popular option for easing the symptoms of gas, indigestion, and bloating. The compound menthol, which is extracted from the peppermint plant, relaxes the muscles in the digestive system and may help ease the symptoms of irritable bowel syndrome (IBS). Herbal teas with additional digestive properties, such as licorice root, dandelion, and fennel, can help with liver function and reduce inflammation. People can support gut health and have a calming, comforting drinking experience by making therapeutic teas and infusions a part of their routine.

**Mocktails and Elixirs for Gut Health:**

Gut-healthy mocktails and elixirs are a tasty and nourishing non-alcoholic substitute for classic cocktails for individuals who prefer them without alcohol. These drinks are made with components that are carefully chosen for their beneficial effects on digestion, like fermented fruits, probiotic-rich kombucha, and herbs that are proven to soothe the gut. The fermented tea beverage known as kombucha has good bacteria that may aid in reestablishing the equilibrium of the gut microbiota, improving digestion and general health. Fermented fruits, such as pineapple or berries, contribute naturally occurring sweetness and extra probiotics and digestive enzymes to improve gut health. In addition to adding flavor, herbs like cinnamon and turmeric have anti-inflammatory qualities that help with digestion. People can make delectable mocktails and elixirs that not only tempt the taste senses but also promote optimal gut health by combining these ingredients in novel ways.

drinks contribute significantly to the preservation of healthy gut flora and provide a tasty and pleasurable means of promoting digestion and general well-being.

People can prioritize their digestive health in a variety of ways, such as by indulging in therapeutic teas and infusions, gut-friendly mocktails and elixirs, or refreshing drinks infused with flavors that are friendly to the gut. People can nourish their bodies from the inside out, encouraging robust gut flora and optimal well-being, by including these beverages in their daily routine.

# CHAPTER ELEVEN
## MEAL PLANS AND DIFFICULTIES FOR GUT HEALTH

Meal planning becomes a critical component when thinking about a cookbook for gut health. Weekly meal planning with an emphasis on gut health can make a big difference in overall health.

Prebiotics, probiotics, and fermented foods are among the components of these meal plans that promote healthy gut flora. Their goal is to develop a well-balanced diet that supports the health of the gut flora, which can help with immunity, digestion, and nutrition absorption.

**Weekly Menus for Digestive Health**

The staples of weekly meal plans for gut health are usually a range of nutrient-dense foods that promote diverse microbiota. A variety of fruits, vegetables, nutritious grains, lean meats, and healthy fats are frequently included in these diets. Including foods that have undergone fermentation, such as kefir, sauerkraut, kimchi, or yogurt, in the diet plan helps to maintain a healthy gut environment by supplying probiotics.

Foods high in prebiotics, like garlic, onions, leeks, asparagus, and bananas, are also frequently consumed to support the gut's natural beneficial bacteria.

Meal plans for gut health frequently include particular foods along with an emphasis on moderation and balance. They might include suggestions for minimizing processed foods, refined sugars, and artificial additives, all of which have been shown to have a deleterious effect on gut health, as well as advice for portion sizes. People may make sure they're regularly eating a range of gut-friendly foods throughout the week, supporting a thriving microbiome and general wellness, by adhering to a well-structured meal plan.

**Particular Food Requirements and Gut Health**

Taking unique dietary requirements into account is essential when creating a cookbook for intestinal health. Many people have dietary needs or preferences that need to be met, such as vegetarian or vegan diets, lactose sensitivity, or gluten intolerance. A cookbook on gut health ought to provide modifications and alternatives to meet these requirements while upholding the fundamentals of encouraging a balanced gut flora.

Recipes utilizing gluten-free grains like quinoa, brown rice, and buckwheat can be added for those who are intolerant to gluten. Recipes using dairy substitutes like almond milk, coconut yogurt, or cashew cheese are beneficial for those who are lactose intolerant. To guarantee sufficient nutrient intake, vegetarian and vegan options might include plant-based protein sources such as beans, lentils, tofu, and tempeh in addition to a range of fruits, vegetables, nuts, and seeds.

A gut health cookbook can reach a larger audience and help more people reap the advantages of gut health optimization by offering a variety of recipes that cater to various dietary requirements.

**Overcoming Typical Obstacles to Improve Gut Health**

Despite the advantages of putting gut health first, there may be obstacles in the road. These difficulties can include finding specific ingredients or navigating social settings where there may not be many gut-friendly options. These limitations must be overcome with ingenuity, adaptability, and a determination to put gut health first despite difficulties.

The availability of specialty ingredients needed for dishes that are gut-friendly is a regular problem. Certain probiotic supplements, plants high in prebiotics, and fermented foods might not be easily available everywhere. In these situations, people can look for alternate sources by visiting nearby health food stores or internet merchants. To guarantee quality and freshness, they can also try creating homemade versions of fermented foods like yogurt, kombucha, or pickles.

Maintaining intestinal health when eating out or at social events where food selections could be limited presents another difficulty. In these circumstances, people should concentrate on choosing the healthiest options available, like whole grains, lean meats, and grilled or steamed veggies. To make sure there are appropriate options available, they can also think about bringing a meal that is good for the gut to share or informing the host in advance of their dietary restrictions.

It might be difficult to incorporate gut-friendly practices into daily living, particularly for people who have demanding lives or have hectic schedules. However, incorporating gut-friendly habits can be done smoothly with the right preparation and arrangement. This could entail meal planning and cooking in bulk on the weekends, giving gut-friendly products top priority when grocery shopping, and coming up with quick, yet wholesome, dishes that fit into your hectic workday schedule.

Ultimately, overcoming typical obstacles to a better gut necessitates taking the initiative, being flexible, and being dedicated to treating gut health as a crucial aspect of overall well-being. Through the proactive resolution of these issues and the application of useful techniques, people can effectively achieve optimal gut health and capitalize on the manifold advantages it provides.

# CONCLUSION

The process of comprehending and promoting gut health has involved empowerment and self-discovery. Our journey into the world of fermented foods, probiotic delights, and prebiotic powerhouses has taken us from the basics of gut-healthy cooking to new heights of culinary exploration that not only tantalize the taste senses but also nourish the body from the inside out.

We've explored the colorful world of innovative snacks and sides, nourishing lunches and dinners, gut-healthy breakfasts, and even decadent desserts—all made with carefully selected foods that support our internal ecosystem. We've embraced a holistic approach to eating that celebrates the complex balance of flavors and nutrients required for good gut health through thoughtful meal plans and pleasant beverages.

As we consider the insights learned and the recipes exchanged, let us keep in mind that each meal we prepare offers a chance to promote health and energy. Incorporating gut-friendly foods and cooking methods into our daily routines helps us to create a thriving internal ecosystem that promotes our general well-being and health in addition to nourishing ourselves.

Raise your glasses to the power of health and food, knowing that every thoughtful mouthful brings us one step closer to living a vibrant, well-being-filled existence. Cheers to the adventure of providing our bodies with nourishment, one delectable meal at a time.